★ ALL ABOUT ★
HORSES

A Kid's Guide to Breeds, Care, Riding, and More!

Kelly Milner Halls

Illustrations by Jessie Willow Tucker

ROCKRIDGE
PRESS

For general information on our other products and services or to obtain technical support, please contact our Customer Care Department within the United States at (866) 744-2665, or outside the United States at (510) 253-0500.

Rockridge Press publishes its books in a variety of electronic and print formats. Some content that appears in print may not be available in electronic books, and vice versa.

Interior and Cover Designer: Lindsey Dekker
Art Producer: Tom Hood
Editor: Laura Apperson
Production Manager: Holly Haydash
Production Editor: Melissa Edeburn

Illustration © Jessie Willow Tucker, 2021

Hardcover ISBN: 978-1-63878-589-7 | Paperback ISBN: 978-1-64739-362-5
eBook ISBN: 978-1-64739-363-2
R0

🐴

This book is dedicated to my adopted wild mustang, Little Bit. She became a tame horse with a wild heart, just for me.

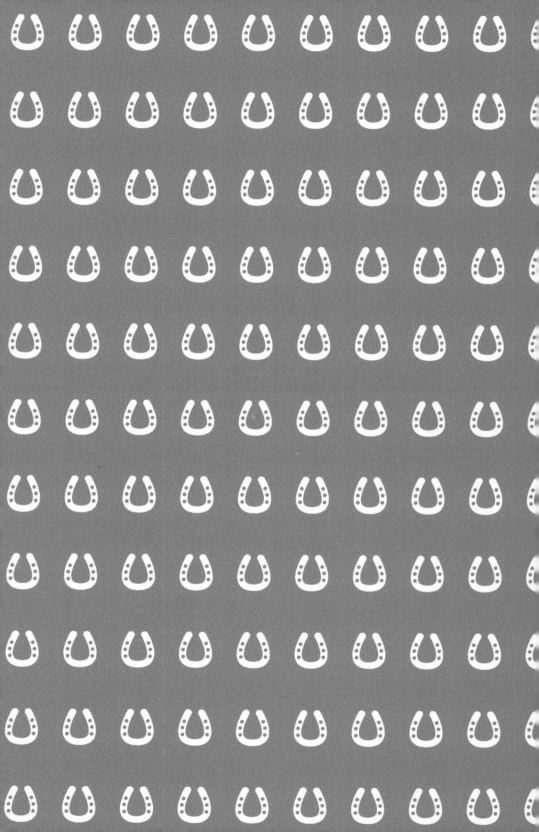

CONTENTS

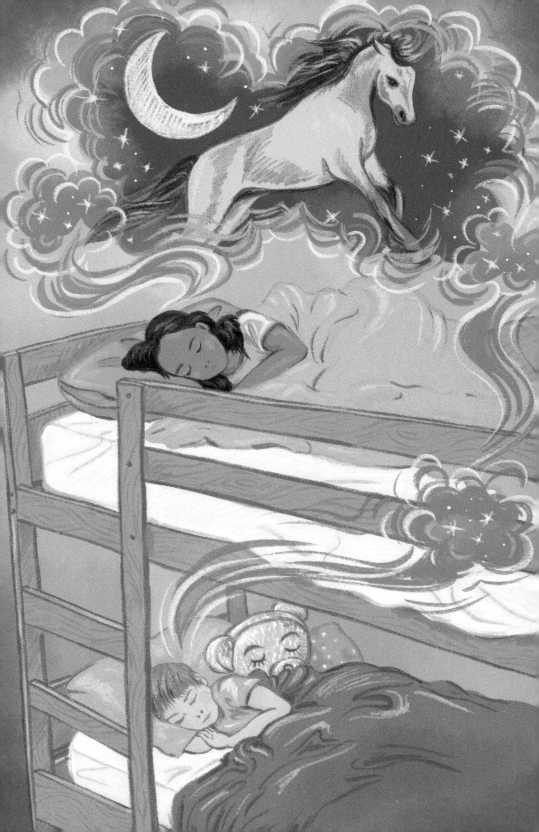

CHAPTER 1

ALL ABOUT HORSES

Do you ever dream of a horse? Do you imagine the sounds it makes? Would you love to brush its mane, ride on its back, or wrap your arms around its neck?

If you answered yes to any of these questions, you may have horse fever. But don't worry—reading this book will make the best of your condition!

You'll get to know the world of horses in this book. You'll learn what they eat, when they sleep, and how they think. Best of all, you'll learn the secret all horse owners discover: The horse you love might learn to love you right back.

THE BASICS

The first horse, Hyracotherium, appeared 55 million years ago in North America. But it was much smaller than horses we see today. Just ten inches high at their shoulders and less than two feet long, Hyracotherium galloped through forests in herds. They feasted on tender leaves and stood on three-hooved toes.

In time, horses **evolved** into the creatures we know and love today. First, they thrived as wild animals, munching grass instead of leaves. In the past as in the present, one powerful male called a stallion leads each wild herd. He commands about 20 adult females called mares, younger males and females, and babies called foals.

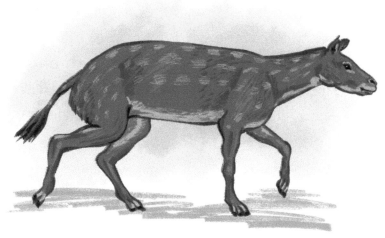

Hyracotherium was the first horse.

Moving from grassland to grassland, horse herds wandered from North America to other continents worldwide. Small horses, called ponies, evolved where grass was hard to find.

For centuries, people hunted horses as meat. But they discovered horses were more valuable as **domesticated**, or tamed, companions about 6,000 years ago. Today, more than two million people love their domesticated horses.

HORSING AROUND Why does a male horse whinny? *To find out "whinny" can eat dinner!*

HORSE STUDY

Many kinds of prehistoric horses once roamed the earth. But only two survived. Scientists call the domesticated horse *Equus caballus*. The second horse is known as *Equus przewalskii*—the Przewalskii horse. Closely related to prehistoric horses seen in 20,000-year-old cave paintings in France and Spain, the Przewalskii horse is very special and very rare. Zebras, donkeys, and mules are the horse's **equine** cousins.

Horses are measured in hands because our ancestors did not have measuring tapes. They used their hands to measure their horses instead. The distance between the bottom of a man's pinky finger to the top of his pointing finger was about four inches. So, one hand equals four inches.

Adult horses that measure under 14 hands from the ground to the shoulders are called ponies. Those that measure 14 hands and above are officially horses.

Though their heights differ, horses and ponies share most physical traits. They all have tender noses, called muzzles, that enjoy human touch. Their eyes are lined with long, fluttering lashes. Their ears turn to hear warnings. Their hooves and coats need constant **grooming**, meaning they must be

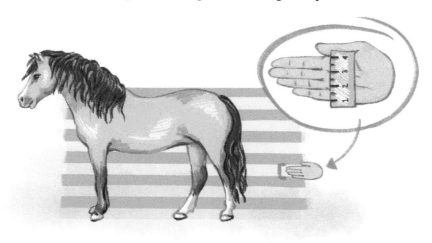

One hand equals four inches.

cleaned to stay healthy. And both ponies and horses need good food, shelter, and medicine.

IN THE SADDLE **Where did scientists first see drawings of prehistoric horses like the Przewalskii?**

A HORSE'S LIFE

When a horse is born, it is called a foal. A girl foal is called a filly and a boy foal is called a colt.

Foals are born hungry, so they search for their mother's milk right away. The milk is full of vitamins and minerals to help the baby fight off sickness.

Within a week, the babies eat grass along with their mother's milk. Within three or four months, they stop drinking milk and start eating more like a grown-up horse.

They are curious but afraid of their human care-takers. Patience and kindness win them over. Soon, they learn to wear their **halters** and follow their humans and their mothers.

Twelve-month-old horses, called yearlings, are too young to ride, and a little too adventurous. They need gentle training to help them learn. Some colts are fixed as yearlings to quiet their instinct to mate. Those males are then called geldings.

Long walks help the yearlings, two-year-olds, and three-year-olds trust their humans. Trust makes riding possible as the

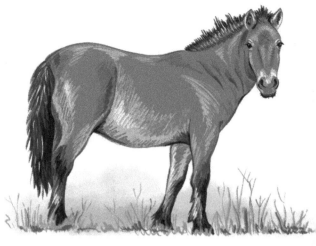

The Przewalskii horse was found in cave paintings.

three-year-olds mature. Smart owners build a loving bond gently—a bond that will last the horse's lifetime. Most horses love their owners in return as a result.

TRUE TAILS: SEFTON THE SOLDIER SURVIVOR

A horse named Sefton was helping with the Changing of the Guard in London, England, on July 20, 1982, when car bombs exploded. Eight horses were hurt, but Sefton had the worst injuries. Veterinarians treated his 34 wounds and gave Sefton a fifty-fifty chance of surviving. He pulled through and was named "Horse of the Year."

TAKE THE QUIZ!

If You Were a Wild Horse, What Member
of the Herd Would You Be?

1. Where do you run in the herd?

a. Out front.

b. Anywhere is fine.

c. Depends on my mood.

d. In the back.

2. How much grass do you eat?

a. Enough to be strong.

b. Enough to feed my babies.

c. I eat when I eat.

d. A little with milk.

3. How do you sleep?

a. Standing up, on guard.

b. Curled up with little ones.

c. Any place will do.

d. Next to mom.

4. Do you like to play?

a. I play with the mares.

b. I play carefully.

c. I play or I fight.

d. I play until I get scared.

If you answered mostly As: You're a stallion.

If you answered mostly Bs: You're a mare.

If you answered mostly Cs: You're a yearling.

If you answered mostly Ds: You're a foal.

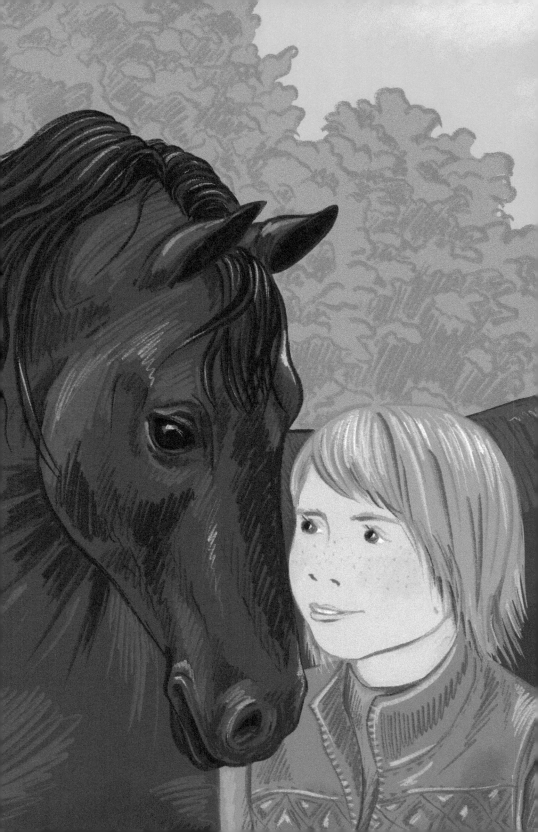

CHAPTER 2

HORSE BEHAVIOR

Talking to horses is fun. But do they understand what we say? Can they talk back? And is there any way to understand what they are saying? Can you know what they are thinking? Can we tell why they do the things they do? Most horse experts say the answer to all these questions is YES. Horses and people can connect in very special ways. This chapter will explain how horses communicate and share their feelings. And if you pay close attention, you may learn what to do and say when you meet a horse, too.

STRAIGHT FROM THE HORSE'S MOUTH

Horses communicate with sounds. If you know what each sound means, you can have a conversation.

Groan

If a horse groans from its belly, it doesn't feel good. It might have a sick stomach or a sore leg. Take it easy if your horse groans.

Nicker

This sound is soft and happy. A horse nickers when it's time for dinner or another fun activity.

Scream

A horse scream is a battle cry. If a horse screams, a fight could happen.

Sigh

Like people, horses sigh when they are relaxed or bored. Brush a horse—happy sigh. Make it stand in one place too long—bored sigh.

Snort

When a horse forces air through its nose, it's called a snort. This sound means the horse is either happy or fearful.

Squeal

A squeal is a horse's way of warning another horse, "Don't come too close."

Whinny/Neigh

This loud sound has two meanings. A happy horse whinnies. A fearful horse neighs.

HORSING AROUND **What do you call a sad horse story?** *A tale of "whoa."*

WATCH OUT FOR BODY LANGUAGE

Horses use sounds to communicate. But how they move, their body language, can say even more. Learn how to read that language, and you will unlock even more horse secrets.

Head

A lowered head means a horse is relaxed and happy. A head held high is worried about something it sees. A head moving from side to side is a warning: Stay away or fight.

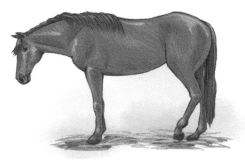

This Thoroughbred horse might be relaxed or happy.

Ears

A horse's ears reflect its feelings. If the ears are forward, the horse is alert. If they are relaxed to the side, the horse might be asleep. If they are turned back and flat against the horse's head, it's angry.

Teeth

If a horse licks its teeth or lips, it's happy. If it bares its teeth, it is either trying to smell something or it is ready to bite.

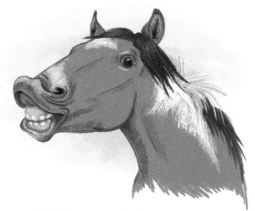

This horse might be trying to smell something or be ready to bite!

Legs

If one back leg is cocked, meaning one foot is slightly off the ground, the horse is relaxed. If a horse paws the ground softly, it's bored. If it strikes hard, it's fighting an enemy. If it kicks its back legs, it's defensive or afraid.

IN THE SADDLE If you see a horse with its head down, what does it mean?

AMAZING ANIMALS

Horses are big, beautiful mammals. They are smart and thoughtful, but every horse has its own special personality.

Wild horses live to eat and to create new members of their herds. They work together to stay safe. But horses trained by good human caregivers can learn to do much more.

Large breeds like the Clydesdales and the Shires are called coldbloods, or heavy horses. They were once used in war, but today they help with farming. They are strong, gentle animals almost anyone could ride.

Hotbloods, or light horses, are not built for hard work. They are made to be fast and full of energy. Arabians and Thoroughbreds are popular light horse breeds. They bond with humans, but they can be stubborn. Riders must work harder to train hotblood breeds.

Horses like the American Quarter Horse or the Tennessee Walker are called warmblooded horses. They are smaller than coldbloods and less stubborn than hotbloods. They are perfect for work on cattle or sheep ranches.

You'll learn more about all three types of horses in chapter 4.

TRUE TAILS: MISTER ED

In the 1960s, Mister Ed was a television show about a man named Wilbur and his talking horse, named Ed. The palomino's real name was Bamboo Harvester, and he had fans worldwide. His favorite treat was sweet tea and hay.

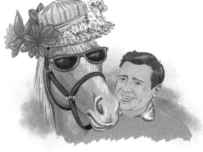

TAKE THE QUIZ!

What Is Your Horse Telling You?

1. Your horse's ears are . . .

a. Facing forward.

b. Floppy.

c. Pinned back.

2. Your horse just . . .

a. Whinnied.

b. Sighed.

c. Screamed.

3. Your horse's leg is . . .

a. Still.

b. Cocked.

c. Pawing the ground hard.

4. Your horse's teeth . . .

a. Are being licked by the horse's tongue.

b. Are bared with the upper lip curled.

c. Are bared with ears pinned.

5. Your horse's head is . . .

a. Not high or low.

b. Low.

c. Swaying from side to side.

Mostly As: Your horse is alert and ready to go.

Mostly Bs: Your horse is happy and relaxed.

Mostly Cs: Your horse is unhappy or angry.

If you have an even mix of As, Bs, and Cs: You've discovered a horse can have many moods at once.

CHAPTER 3

HORSE TRAITS

Most horses belong to the same family of animals, and yet, they can look very different. Some are large and strong. They do heavy work and were once used for battle. Some are small but determined. They live in climates that might be hard on other horses.

Some horses are brown in color. Some are dark with splashes of white. Some have a golden glow.

They move differently, too. Some are slow, but steady. Others love to race across an open prairie.

This chapter will explore these amazing differences. It might help you decide which horse would be perfect—just for you.

PATTERNS, COATS & MARKINGS

All horses have coats of hair that are thick in the winter to keep them warm. But as the temperature warms, a horse's coat changes.
By midsummer, it is thin, smooth, and shiny.
   All horses have this coat change in common. But their colors and markings can be very different. Horse experts have created names for groups with special colors and markings.

- Appaloosas look like they've been splattered with small, dark spots.

- Bay and brown horses have brown coats with black manes and tails.

- Black horses have dark black coats, manes, and tails.

- Buckskin and dun horses have light brown coats with black manes and tails.

- Chestnut horses have red-brown coats with matching manes and tails.

- Cremello horses have pale golden coats with white manes and tails.

- Gray horses have gray coats with black manes and tails.

- Paint horses have large patches of white, brown, or black.

- Palomino horses are yellow with white manes and tails.

HORSE SENSE

Horses seem to have the same senses people have—sight, sound, smell, taste, and touch. But their senses work differently from ours.

Sight

People and other meat eaters have eyes on the front of their faces. Plant eaters like horses have eyes on the sides of their heads. They see from two directions at once. But they have a blind spot in front.

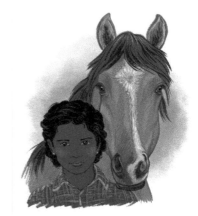

A rider and their Quarter Horse look straight ahead.

Sound

Horses also hear from two directions at once. Each ear can turn to detect two different sounds, like a snake *and* a footstep, before people hear them.

Smell

A horse's sense of smell is more powerful than ours. They can smell friends and enemies from a distance, and they smell food long before they see it.

Taste

Horses have **taste buds** on their tongues and the roofs of their mouths. They love the taste of many foods.

Touch

A horse's whole body is as sensitive as a human's fingertip. They can feel things like a fly, a brush, a metal mouthpiece, or pressure from a rider's leg.

IN THE SADDLE A horse's sense of touch is more sensitive than ours, but they sometimes ignore human signals. Why?

GAITS & GALLOPS

Watching a horse move is magical. Every horse has its own grace and strength. But they all naturally move in five different ways, called gaits.

Walk

A walk is a relaxed, four-beat gait used to graze for grass or gently wander. It is a horse's slowest gait, at four miles per hour.

Trot

A trot is a faster, two-beat pattern gait. The horse's legs work in pairs. It has a bounce to it at about eight miles per hour.

Canter

A canter is a rolling, three-beat gait. It is faster and smoother than a trot, but it is not the fastest gait at 12 to 15 miles per hour.

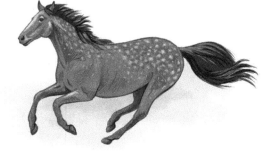

Gallop

The gallop looks like a fast canter, but it is actually a four-beat

This Thoroughbred is in a gallop.

gait. At times, a horse at a full gallop is airborne, but only for a second or two. A gallop covers 25 to 40 miles per hour.

Back Up

When a horse backs up in a two-beat gait, it's a careful way to escape a narrow space. It can be a very slow gait.

TRUE TAILS: SHADOWFAX

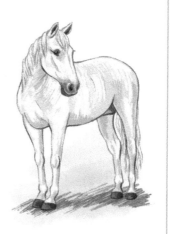

When J. R. R. Tolkien wrote his *Lord of the Rings* stories, he created Shadowfax, lord of all horses. Gandalf the wise wizard could speak to the silvery Andalusian stallion. Shadowfax sometimes carried Gandalf across **Middle Earth**, as fast as the wind.

TAKE THE QUIZ!

If You Were a Horse, Which Gait Might Be Your Favorite?

1. When you're late to school you . . .

a. Take it easy.

b. Hurry a little.

c. Race your brother.

d. Beat everyone to the car.

e. Go back to bed.

2. When you smell dinner, you . . .

a. Go to the table, eventually.

b. Wonder what's cooking.

c. Hope for your favorite food.

d. Help put it on the table.

e. Wait for your parents to call you.

3. At the school dance, you . . .

a. Like slow dances.

b. Hope for a pop song.

c. Love disco.

d. Bounce to punk.

e. Go home early.

4. When homework is calling, you . . .

a. Get it done by bedtime.

b. Do it in time to watch TV.

c. Do it right after school.

d. Finish it in class.

e. Do it before breakfast.

Mostly As: You're a walker.

Mostly Bs: You're a trotter.

Mostly Cs: Canter's your vibe.

Mostly Ds: Gallop on.

Mostly Es: You back up!

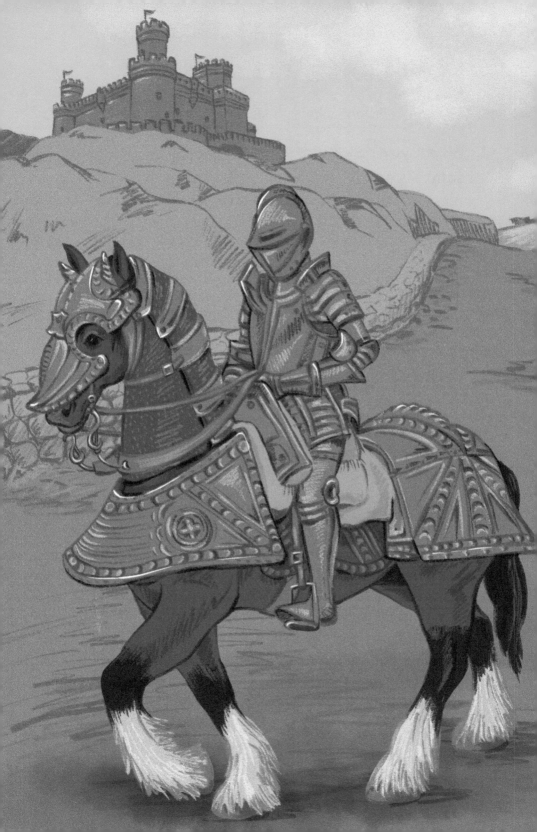

CHAPTER 4

HORSE TYPES

In chapter 3, we explored groups that describe what horses look like. In this chapter, we'll explore groups that describe how they act. Coldbloods, hotbloods, and warmbloods are those groups.

The coldbloods are easygoing by nature. They are relaxed and easy to work with. The hotbloods are fast and alert. They have spirit and can be hard to ride without experience. The warmbloods fall right in the middle. They can be fast and lively, but if they trust a human, they cooperate.

Which horses fall into each of the three categories? You'll soon find out.

COLDBLOODS

Coldbloods are the gentle giants of the horse world. Two hands and 200 pounds larger than most other horses, they have enough strength for farming, logging, or pulling heavy wagons.

Coldbloods were war horses many years ago. They were able to carry the weight of a large man, even when he wore a 50-pound suit of armor. It was a dangerous job. But a well-trained horse was valuable. Knights tried to protect their giant horses.

With thicker coats, manes, tails, and even tufts of hair at their ankles, coldbloods do well in frosty weather. They are not often used for riding today, but they are bright and gentle. Their owners appreciate them.

Some coldblood breeds, like the Black Forest, the Rhenish German, and the Austrian Noriker, are disappearing. Tractors have replaced these draft horses on most farms. But their biggest fans are trying to save them.

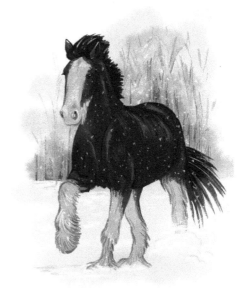

Clydesdales can live in cold climates.

A few coldblood breeds are still very popular. The American Cream Draft, the Belgian, the Clydesdale, the Percheron, and the Shire are all work horses and show horses.

HORSING AROUND Why was the warmblood horse named Goldilocks? *Because she was just right.*

HOTBLOODS

Hotblood horses are not extra-large. But their personalities are huge. Prized for their ability to race across the desert sands of the Middle East, they are light, smart, and very strong-willed.

The graceful Arabian is one of the oldest hot-blood breeds on earth. They have beautiful dished (meaning softly curved) faces and lively, prancing movements. Arabians carry their silky tails high when they are excited.

Today, Arabian horses are popular as show horses and trail horses. They can be hard to ride, but an Arabian that trusts its rider is unstoppable.

Thoroughbreds are another kind of hotblood horse. Thanks to their speed and competitive nature, Thoroughbreds are often racehorses. They want to cross the finish line first.

Thoroughbreds also make excellent show horses for experienced riders. Their long legs and determination are perfect for leaping over **jumps**. And crowds love to watch them perform **dressage**, a dance-like series of movements.

Other hotblood horses include the Akhal-Teke, a cousin to the Arabian, the Spanish Andalusian, and the Barb, originally from North Africa.

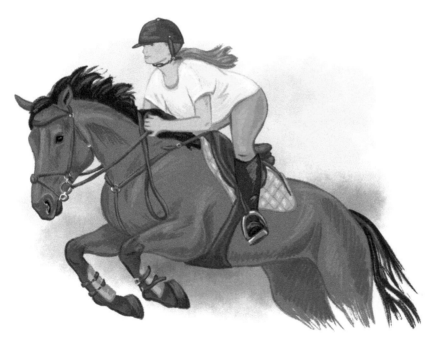

This Thoroughbred is in a jump.

WARMBLOODS

Horse lovers see things in coldbloods and hot-bloods that they really like. So experts created a whole new group—the warmbloods. By mating a coldblood with a hotblood, they created horses that were a little of both.

Warmblood horses have the easygoing attitude of a coldblood *and* the endurance, or the ability to keep going for a long time, of a hotblood. They have the strength of a hotblood *and* the determination of a coldblood. Some say they are the best of both worlds.

The Lipizzan is a warmblood breed. It is known for its muscular body *and* its athletic gaits. One group of Lipizzan stallions trained in Vienna, Austria, is famous. Thanks to the trust between horse and rider, they perform the **equestrian** dance of dres-sage for audiences worldwide.

Quarter horses are another friendly warmblood breed. Ranchers mated Thoroughbred hotbloods with wild horses tamed by the Chickasaw tribe to create this breed. They became fast, stocky, intelligent animals—perfect for work or play.

Other popular warmbloods include the Morgan, the Holsteiner, the Hanoverian, and the Tennessee Walker.

TRUE TAILS: SECRETARIAT

Thoroughbred racehorse Secretariat was famous for winning the Triple Crown, three famous American horse races, on June 10, 1973. His heart weighed 22 pounds. It was more than twice the size of an average Thoroughbred heart. Carrots were his favorite snack.

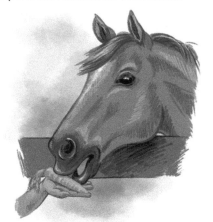

TAKE THE QUIZ!

Which "Blood" Is the Best Horse for You?

1. Your favorite hobby is . . .

a. Chess.

b. Golf.

c. Soccer.

2. Your favorite meal is . . .

a. Breakfast.

b. Lunch.

c. Dinner.

3. Your favorite pop star is . . .

a. Ed Sheeran.

b. Harry Styles.

c. Lizzo.

4. Your favorite Winnie-the-Pooh character is . . .

a. Eeyore.

b. Pooh.

c. Tigger.

5. Your favorite kind of TV show is . . .

a. The news.

b. Cartoons.

c. Basketball.

6. Your favorite snack is . . .

a. Carrot sticks.

b. Cheese.

c. Candy.

Mostly As: You'd like a coldblood.

Mostly Bs: You'd like a warmblood.

Mostly Cs: You'd like a hotblood.

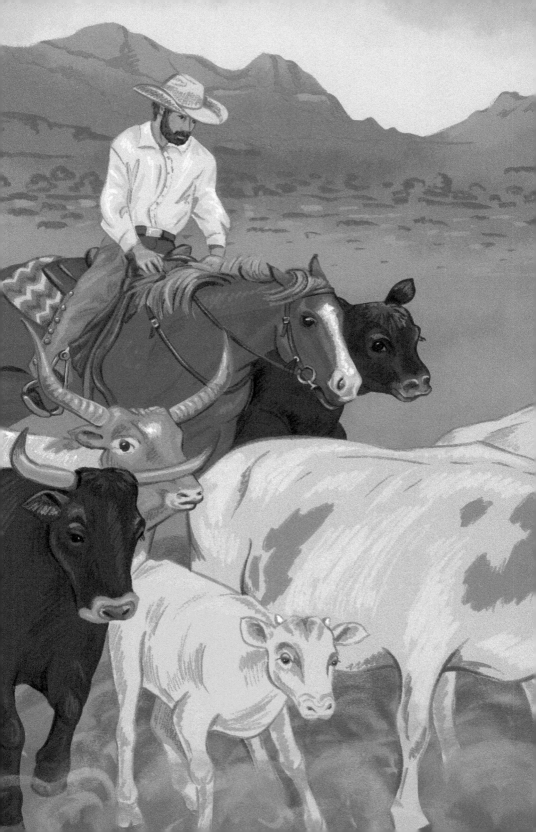

CHAPTER 5

HORSE BREEDS

Prehistoric horses had a certain look thousands of years ago. But as they wandered to new parts of the world, they adapted, or changed as needed. If it was too cold, they grew thicker coats. If it was hot, they became sleek and lean.

When human beings tamed horses, they liked how some looked more than others. If they really liked a certain look, they would mate two horses with the same general look. They were hoping to create a foal that looked like its parents.

Those special looks became horse breeds, including coldbloods, hotbloods, warmbloods, and ponies.

COLDBLOODED BREEDS

Often called draft horses, here are three popular, intelligent coldblood breeds:

Clydesdale

Named for the River Clyde in Scotland, Clydesdales came to North America in the 1800s. They are 16 to 18 hands high and weigh 1,600 pounds or more. Many are bays with white tufts of hair on their ankles, called fringe, and white markings, called blazes, on their faces.

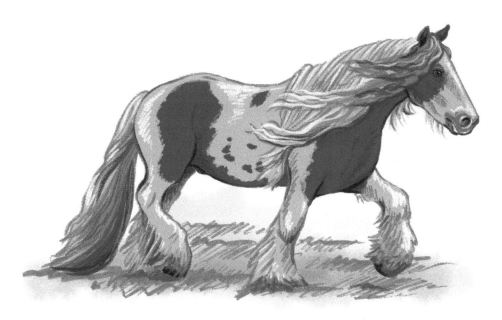

Clydesdale horses are big and strong but very gentle.

Shire

Shire horses are between 16 and 18 hands high and have fringe on their feet. But the British-bred black-, brown-, or gray-coated horses are heavier than Clydesdales at 1,800 to 2,400 pounds. Their ancestors carried soldiers in ancient wars.

Belgian

Europe's Belgian horses were once called Flanders horses. They are very muscular, with little to no foot fringe. Bay and browns were popular in the past, but **sorrels**, with reddish-brown coats and blond manes and tails, are popular Belgians today.

HORSING AROUND Why did cave painters draw horses? *They wanted to horse around.*

HOTBLOODED BREEDS

Hotblooded horses are smaller and leaner than coldbloods. Here are three of the most popular:

Arabian

Arabian horses came from the Middle East thousands of years ago. Considered small at 15 hands tall and 1,000 pounds, Arabians were preferred by histor- ical figures like the prophet Mohammed and George Wash- ington. Gray and bay Arabians are the most popular.

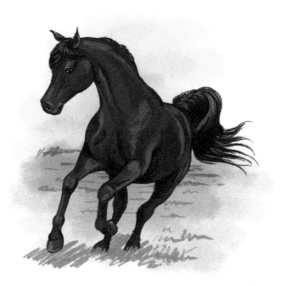

This Arabian horse has a dark coat.

Spanish Barb

When Spanish explorers set out to conquer the world, they brought Spanish Barb horses with them. The small (14-hand), sturdy champions became the favorite of Indigenous tribes in North America. These horses roam American deserts and are known as "wild" horses today.

Thoroughbred

Thoroughbreds are best known as racehorses. But the large (16-hand), lean horses make excellent show and pleasure horses, too. Because of their fiery nature, Thoroughbreds form strong friendships with more experienced riders.

WARMBLOODED BREEDS

By mating hotbloods with coldbloods, the warmbloods were created. These are three of the most popular warmblood breeds:

American Quarter Horse

In the 1800s, American cowboys raised cattle. The smart and sturdy American quarter horse helped move the herds. Between 14 and 16 hands and from 950 to 1,200 pounds, they are faithful companions.

Morgan

The Morgan was bred by a teacher in Massachusetts in the 1700s. The small (14 to 15 hands, 900 to 1,100 pounds) horses are famous for their great personalities. They come in almost all colors and patterns.

Tennessee Walker

Created in the United States, the Tennessee Walker is known for its unusual gaits. It has a regular walk, a running walk, a trot, and a canter. They can be 14 to 17 hands tall, between 900 and 1,200 pounds, and come in virtually all colors.

IN THE SADDLE Why would smaller horses do better in dry, desert climates? How would being small help them survive?

PONY BREEDS

Ponies are the smallest of horses. Here are two popular breeds and a bonus miniature horse:

Shetland

Shetland ponies, from Scotland, are the smallest breed of pony at just 40 inches high. Shetland ponies were pack animals on roads and in mines before they became popular for children to ride. They are sturdy and come in most colors and patterns.

Welsh

These ponies have Arabian blood and are larger and leaner because of it. Welsh ponies once worked on farms and in mines, but today they are popular for smaller riders. They are between 12 and 15 hands high.

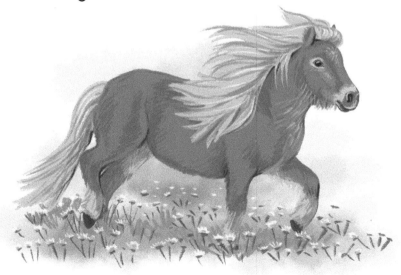

Shetland ponies are the smallest breed of pony.

Miniature Horse

Miniature horses are not ponies, but they are pony-sized. They are no more than 34 inches tall and weigh in between 150 and 250 pounds. They are not thick like ponies. They look like full-size horses hit with a shrink ray. Most miniature horses are not ridden. They are pets and show horses, and they come in most colors and patterns.

TRUE TAILS: THREE BARS

Three Bars was born a Thoroughbred colt in Kentucky in 1940. Although he was raised to run in one-mile to mile-and-a-half races, injuries held him back. But when a new owner bought him to improve the quarter horse breed, his foals and grand-foals became racing champions on the shorter quarter-mile horse races.

TAKE THE QUIZ!

Which Horse Is Best for Your Lifestyle?

1. What do you want?

a. I do not want to ride.

b. I want to ride trails.

c. I want to jump fences.

d. I want to drive a wagon.

2. What color horse is your favorite?

a. Any color will do.

b. I like brown and patterned horses.

c. I like brown and gray horses.

d. I like horses with white, furry feet.

3. How much do you want to feed your horse?

a. A little.

b. Enough.

c. Lots of high-energy food.

d. Tons of food.

Mostly As: You might want a miniature horse.

Mostly Bs: You might like a Morgan or a quarter horse.

Mostly Cs: How about an Arabian?

Mostly Ds: A draft horse may be in your future.

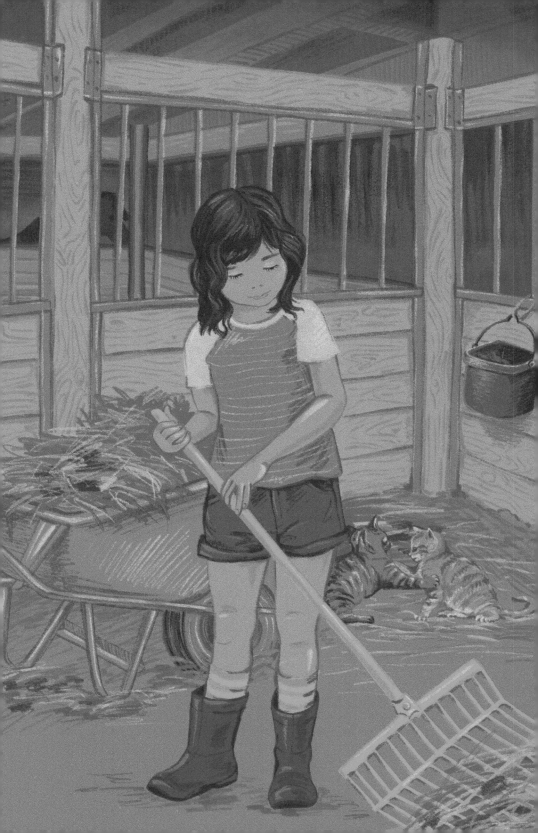

CHAPTER 6

HORSE CARE

Loving horses is easy. Taking care of a horse is a little bit harder. Horses in the wild take care of their own needs. But horses kept by human beings need help. Domesticated horses need a safe place to live. They need plenty of healthy food to eat and clean water to drink. Horses need to be groomed and exercised almost every day. And horses need medical care from veterinarians.

This chapter will guide you through what it takes to own a horse. The hard work you put in will make your horse one of the best friends you'll ever have.

HAY IS FOR HORSES

In the wild, horses eat plants growing on open land. Horses kept by people need the same nutrients.

A **pastured** horse can eat 20 pounds of plants in a single day. A horse that grazes eight hours a day will eat six or seven pounds, only a third of what it needs. Humans need to make up the difference using hay—plants grown on farms and gathered into rectangles called bales.

Alfalfa hay is popular because it is high in protein and vitamins, but clover, oat, barley, and Bermuda hays are also used as food. An average horse eats 50 to 75 bales of hay every year.

Hardworking horses also need grain. A mix of oats, barley, and corn with vitamin and mineral pellets works for active horses. A splash of molasses sweetens the mix, but not too much. Sugar is bad for horses, but a carrot or an apple slice is fine for a daily treat.

Don't forget fresh water. Horses drink five to 10 gallons a day.

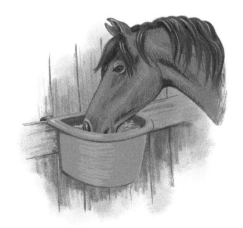

A Spanish Barb horse eats from its feeding bin.

HAIRCARE & GROOMING

To groom your horse properly, you need the right tools.

Brushes

Dandy brushes have stiff bristles to remove mud from a horse's coat. Body brushes are softer for dust and skin cells. Curry combs are oval rubber brushes used to remove dust and shed hair.

Clippers and Scissors

Use clippers and scissors to trim a horse's hair, but never the hairs around a horse's eye and muzzle. Those hairs protect horses from getting too close to sharp objects. If you don't clip your horse's mane and tail, you might braid or band them for special events.

Hoof Pick

Hoof picks remove mud, rocks, and bacteria from the bottom of a horse's foot.

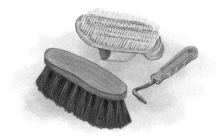

Clockwise from bottom left: dandy brush, curry comb, hoof pick.

Mane and Tail Comb

This comb helps detangle the mane and tail.

Rags and Sponges

Gentle rags and sponges clean a horse's eyes and ears.

Shampoo

Horses rarely need a bath, but sometimes they might need a wash before a show or special occasion.

Shoes

Some horses need metal shoes; some don't. An expert called a **farrier** knows what is best for each horse.

STABLE LIFE

People keep their horses at home or board them at a stable for a monthly fee, like rent.

If you pay a lot, the stable takes care of all your horse's needs. If you pay less, you do some of the work.

That work starts at dawn when the horses start to whinny. Filling their bellies is the first chore. You'll need to clean the feed bins, then add a little hay and a little grain. Soon, you'll hear nothing but *crunch, crunch, crunch.*

Next, clean the water troughs and fill them to the brim with fresh water.

After the horses are fed and watered, turn them outside. Some go to big pastures. Some go to small **paddocks**.

While the horses are outside, clean the stalls. This job is sometimes called mucking out the stalls. Horses go to the bathroom at night. If you don't clean it up, the horses can get sick.

Rake up the dirty bedding, shovel it into a wheelbarrow, and dump it on the stable dung hill—the pile of waste from the horses' stalls. In time, that waste will become fertilizer.

Add fresh straw, wood shavings, or wood pellets to the clean floors and the stall is ready for the night. As the sun sets, the horses whinny again. Time for dinner and a safe night in the stalls.

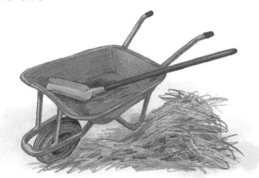

TRUE TAILS: BLACK BEAUTY

Black Beauty isn't a real horse, but she is a legend. Created by writer Anna Sewell, the story followed how Black Beauty was mistreated. After more than 50 million copies were sold, new laws were written to protect real horses from mistreatment.

TAKE THE QUIZ!

Is It Time to Groom Your Horse?

When it comes to caring for a horse, little things can mean a lot. Take this quiz for a few examples!

1. Your horse's coat looks . . .

a. Smooth and shiny.

b. Dusty and dull.

c. Like it slept in a mud puddle.

2. Your horse's stall is . . .

a. Fresh and clean.

b. Dotted with poo.

c. So stinky you can hardly stand it.

3. Your horse looks . . .

a. Ready to win a blue ribbon.

b. Okay.

c. Too thin.

Mostly As: You're on top of caring for your horse. Keep up the good work.

Mostly Bs: It's time grab your curry comb and a rake to clean things up.

Mostly Cs: It's time to put more food in the bins, groom a little longer, and clean the stall really well.

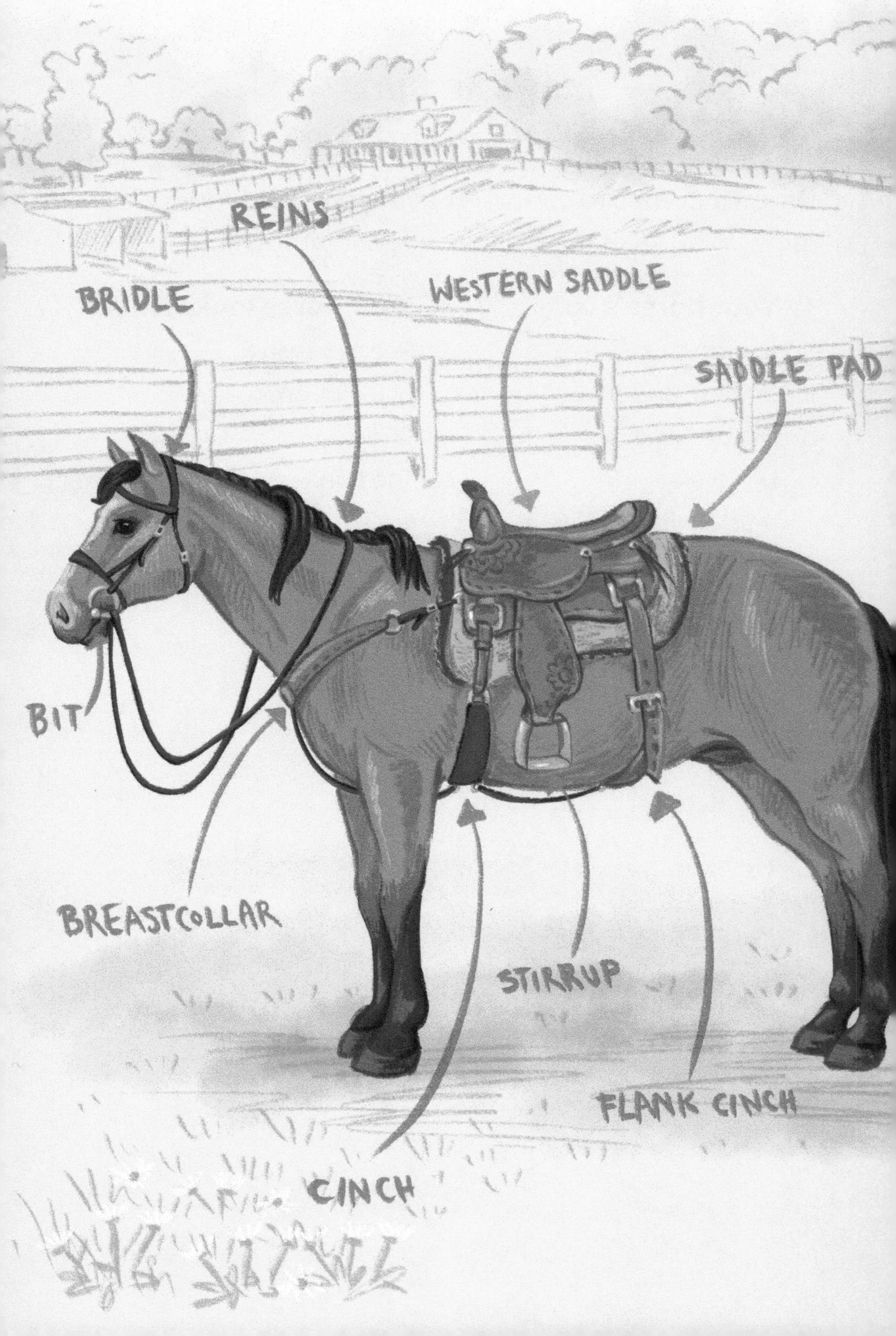

REINS

BRIDLE

WESTERN SADDLE

SADDLE PAD

BIT

BREASTCOLLAR

STIRRUP

FLANK CINCH

CINCH

CHAPTER 7

HORSEBACK RIDING

Watching horses is fun. But riding horses is magical! When a horse trusts a rider, almost anything seems possible. But what does it take to climb in the saddle? How do you learn to work with 1,500 pounds of animal?

This chapter will reveal the secrets to making a horse your partner. You'll learn what tools you need to ride—like saddles, bridles, and cinches. You'll come to understand what makes a horse afraid of you and what makes a horse your friend.

You'll discover why kindness is much better than fear when your best friend is a powerful horse.

RIDING GEAR

When you're ready to climb onto a horse, you'll need all the right equipment.

Riders need:

- Boots with a small heel.

- Sturdy pants like blue jeans that stretch without tearing.

- Comfortable shirts and jackets that don't make too much noise.

- Helmets in case new riders take a tumble.

Horses need their own riding equipment, called **tack**:

- Halters fit on a horse's head with a rope at the bottom to lead the horse from one place to another.

- Saddle blankets protect your horse from the sharp edges of a saddle.

- Saddles fit on a horse's back for riding. A cinch around the horse's belly holds it in place.

- Bridles fit on a horse's head. A metal bit on the bridle slips into the horse's mouth. Bridles replace halters for telling the horse what you want when you're riding.

- Reins, long strips of leather, attach to the bridle and the bit, letting you guide the horse as you ride.

- Breast collars help keep the saddle from slipping, but not everyone uses one.

HORSING AROUND **Why did the horsefly stare at the horse?** *It was jealous.*

GALLOPING TOGETHER

Most riders learn in an arena, a large dirt oval with wooden fencing. Mount the horse from its left side. Stand on your right foot and lift your left foot up to the left **stirrup**. Slip your foot in, grip the saddle with both hands, and raise yourself up to the horse's back.

Gently move your right leg over the horse's back and slip your foot into the right stirrup. Push your heels down and keep them there. Now you're ready to ride.

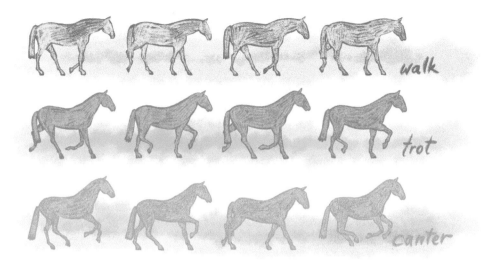

walk

trot

canter

Warm your horse up by walking three or four times around the arena. The walk is the easiest gait for you and your horse.

Move into the bouncy trot—the second gait. You may feel a little out of control. If you ride Western style, relax your stomach muscles and absorb the bounce. If you ride English style, post in the trot, which means to sit and stand to match your horse's rhythm.

Canter is the next gait—a rolling, smooth motion. Gently pull back on your reins and release them to slow down your horse.

If you feel scared, firmly pull back on the reins and say, "Whoa." That will tell the horse to stop.

SAFETY FIRST

Riding a horse is joining forces with another living animal. That means it's important to keep yourself AND the horse safe, and these steps will make that possible.

1. Groom your horse before you **tack up**. Dirt under the saddle can cause a sore.

2. Check for cuts and swelling. If your horse is hurt, ride another day.

3. Check the area for nails before you ride so your horse doesn't get hurt.

4. Don't ride when it's too rainy. Your horse could fall and hurt you both.

5. Don't pull too hard on the reins. It will hurt your horse's mouth.

6. Wear a helmet and keep your heels down in the stirrups.

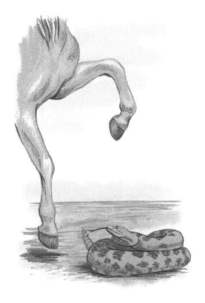

This Arabian horse is avoiding a snake! Check the area before you ride.

7. Don't ride too fast before you're ready.

8. Stay alert. If danger approaches, be ready.

IN THE SADDLE If you pull too hard on the reins, will the bit hurt your horse's mouth?

TRUE TAILS: BROOKLYN SUPREME

Brooklyn Supreme was born in 1928. The sturdy Belgian colt grew to be a huge stallion, one of the biggest horses ever known. He weighed 3,200 pounds and stood 19.2 hands tall. But he was so gentle that kids giggled when he stole their ice cream cones.

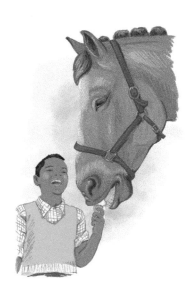

TAKE THE QUIZ!

As a Rider, Which Gait Might You Like Best?

1. **At the amusement park, you like to ride ...**
   a. The carousel.
   b. The bumper cars.
   c. A roller coaster.

2. **Your favorite exercise is ...**
   a. Sit-ups.
   b. Jogging.
   c. Riding a bike.

3. **Your favorite snack is ...**
   a. String cheese.
   b. Jello.
   c. A smoothie.

4. **Your favorite books are ...**
   a. Long.
   b. Short.
   c. Who cares, as long as it's great?

5. **You watch television ...**
   a. All the time.
   b. Now and then.
   c. When the show is action-packed.

Mostly As: Your gait is the walk.

Mostly Bs: Your gait is the trot.

Mostly Cs: Your gait is the canter.

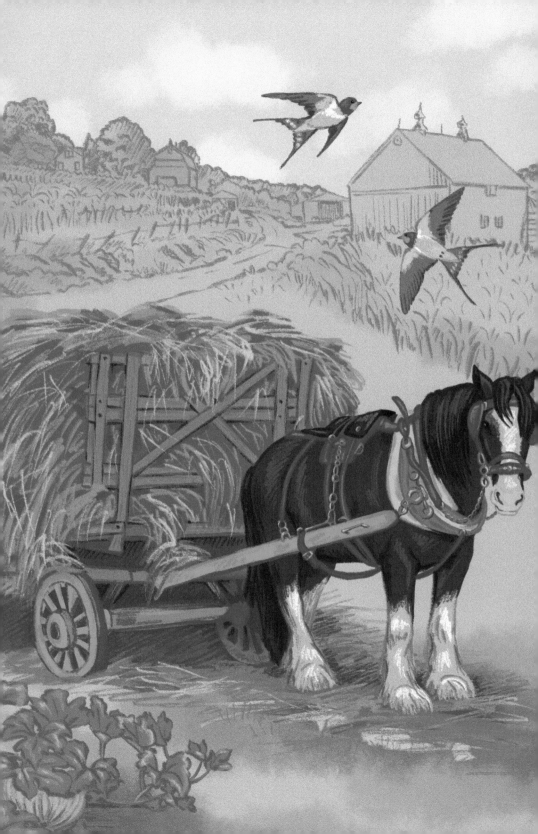

CHAPTER 8

HORSES IN OUR WORLD

For thousands of years, people have treasured horses for the joy of riding. But the noble animals have helped us with our work, too.

Farmers depended on horses to help plant, plow, and harvest food before there were tractors to do those jobs. Horses pulled city wagons, streetcars, and fire engines. They even once pulled trains.

Horses helped soldiers fight against their enemies, long before tanks or trucks or bomber planes existed.

Without horses, the world might not have moved forward. This chapter will explore just how important horses have been to human progress.

HORSES ON THE FARM

Humans began taming horses around 4,000 BCE. At first, they used horses for meat and milk. But they soon realized they were better as animal companions. Horses could help them grow food, too.

The harness, a collar with reins draped around the horse's neck, made it possible for people to use a large horse to move things. If a farmer cleared land of trees and plants to grow crops, but a stone or stump was in the way, a large horse with a harness could remove it.

Soon, farmers discovered that horses could pull more than rocks and trees. They could pull plows and **harrows** to break up the soil, then plant and cover seed. Farming took less time with a good horse.

Thanks to the horse, farmers could grow more food than they needed for their own families. Horses pulled wagons full of the extra harvest to sell in town. Horses helped farmers feed their friends and earn extra money for clothes and household goods

---

HORSING AROUND Why did the farmer stand behind the horse? *He got a kick out of it.*

SERVICE HORSES

Horses bond so closely with people that they can do more than farm. Service horses can help heal human bodies and souls.

Horse therapy may have started with the ancient Greeks. But it really got noticed in 1969 when people realized that riding gentle horses would help people with disabilities improve their lives.

Being outside with a gentle animal, large or small, helped people deal with their pain and their emotional disappointments, especially kids 6 to 18 years old. Being with horses helped ease stress, anger, sadness, and distraction. It also helped kids feel confident and more trusting.

Why are horses good therapists? Because they don't judge people based on what they look like or what they have. Horses trust people based on how they are treated. They remind us how to treat our family and friends, too.

Horses also serve us as four-legged police companions. Big city police officers ride horses to control large

Miniature horses are common service horses.

crowds of people in busy places. The horse's height allows an officer to see over the heads of the people.

Because they work every day on pavement, most police horses either go barefoot—no metal horseshoes—or they wear rubber boots, instead.

IN THE SADDLE **Horses can tell when a person is in a good mood or a bad mood. How could that help them as therapy animals?**

FRIENDS FOREVER

How did we learn thousands of years ago that we could have a real relationship with horses? Maybe a gentle horse took an apple from a young girl's hand, and a friendship was born. Perhaps a boy was hurt far from home, and a wild horse carried him to safety.

However it happened, the connection is real. We may not need horses

Shetland ponies make great friends.

for modern farming or war anymore, but we cherish them as faithful friends.

Building a relationship with a horse takes time. It takes patience and determination. There are good days and bad days, but if you keep trying, it happens. And the connection can last for many, many years.

Most people who spend time with horses believe they are worth the hard work it takes to win them over. And they wouldn't want to live without them.

Sadly, we can't all have horses of our own. But we can all care about them. And we can always hope that someday, our horse dreams will come true.

TRUE TAILS: TRIGGER

Roy Rogers was a famous singing cowboy in the 1930s, '40s, and '50s. But his horse Trigger was the real star. Called the "smartest horse in the movies," the beautiful palomino stallion could perform more than 150 tricks.

TAKE THE QUIZ!

What Kind of Service Horse Are You?

1. What do you do after breakfast?

a. Clear open land of rocks and trees.

b. Slip into rubber boots and other tack.

c. Wait for sad people to visit.

2. Where do you work?

a. On big pieces of land.

b. On busy city streets.

c. At schools and offices.

3. What is your favorite snack?

a. Fresh apples from the farm.

b. Ice cream I sneak from crowds.

c. I like hugs better than snacks.

4. Where do you sleep?

a. In a barn.

b. At the police station.

c. In my little stable.

Mostly As: You're a farm horse!

Mostly Bs: You're a police horse!

Mostly Cs: You're a therapy horse!

EQUINE EXTRA!
HORSE FUN, WITHOUT HORSES

If you love horses but you can't have one, check out today's best model horses. Carefully made to look exactly like real horses, only smaller, high-quality models can be fitted with tiny tack. And you can buy miniature barns, arenas, jumps, ribbons, and grooming tools, too.

Wish you could show a horse? You can! Enter a model horse show, in-person or by mail, with photographs. A real judge will decide if your model is a winner. If it is, you'll get real ribbons, just like regular horse owners collect.

For more information about models and model horse shows, visit the North American Model Horse Shows Association online (Resources, page 71).

You can also check out Breyer Horses, the most famous model makers in the world (Resources, page 71).

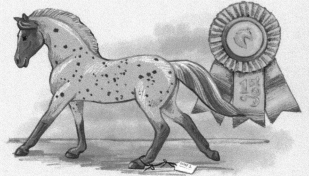

Win a ribbon with your model horse!

TAKE THE BONUS QUIZ!

How Much Do You Love Horses?

1. **If you were a pioneer farmer, you would want a horse . . .**
    a. To help with farming.
    b. To pull the wagon.
    c. To brush and ride.

2. **What kind of horse will you buy?**
    a. A model horse
    b. A horse stuffed animal
    c. A real horse

3. **When you read a horse book, you . . .**
    a. Look at the pictures.
    b. Read the words.
    c. Look at the pictures and read the words.

4. **Your favorite horse is . . .**
    a. A pony.
    b. A draft horse.
    c. A wild mustang.

Mostly As: You REALLY love horses.

Mostly Bs: You REALLY love horses.

Mostly Cs: You REALLY love horses.

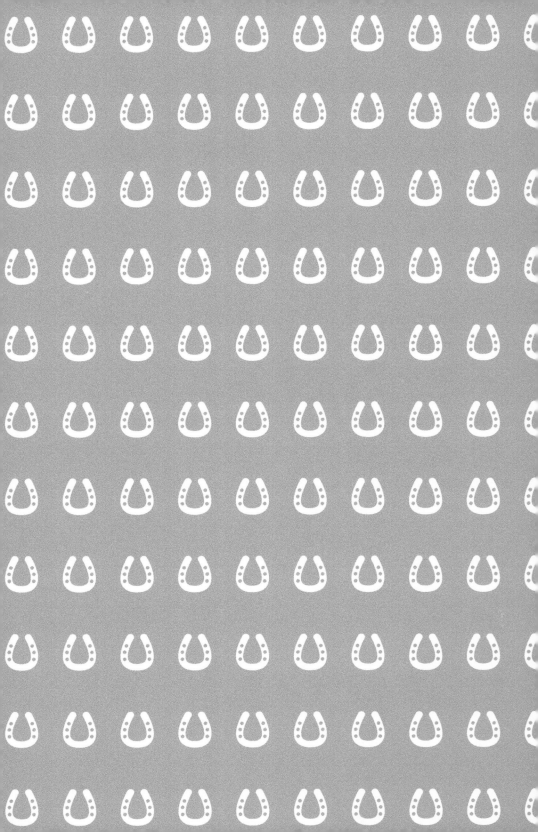

GLOSSARY

domesticated: Tamed by human beings

dressage: A dance-like series of movements performed by a highly trained horse and rider

equestrian: A person who rides or cares for horses

equine: A horse or horse-related item

evolved: Adapted or changed by nature

farrier: A person who cares for a horse's hooves

grooming: The act of brushing, cleaning, and trimming the coats of horses, dogs, or cats

halter: A face-mounted piece of tack used to help control a horse while walking beside it

harrow: A farm tool with teeth used to break up hard dirt

horse therapy: A way to get help with personal problems through caring for and riding gentle horses

jumps: Manmade gates or bars created for horses and riders to leap over in practice arenas and horse shows

Middle Earth: A fictional land created by author J. R. R. Tolkien in his books *The Hobbit* and *The Lord of the Rings*

paddock: A small, fenced place to keep a horse

pasture: A large piece of fenced, grassy land used to keep horses

sorrel: A horse with a reddish-brown coat and light blond mane and tail

stirrups: Metal or wooden loops with flat bottoms that are attached to saddles for a rider's feet

tack: Equipment used to lead and ride a horse

tack up: To put tack on a horse for leading or riding

taste buds: Tiny parts of the tongue that make it possible to taste food

RESOURCES

BOOKS: NONFICTION

Horse: Discover the World of Horses and Ponies by Juliet Clutton-Brock (for readers 8 to 12)

Horse Life: The Ultimate Guide to Caring for and Riding Horses for Kids by Robyn Smith (for readers 8 to 12)

BOOKS: FICTION

Spirit Riding Free: Meet the PALs by Jennifer Fox (for readers 4 to 8)

Summer Pony by Jean Slaughter Doty (for readers 6 to 9)

OTHERS

Breyer Horses: BreyerHorses.com

Identify Your Breyer: IdentifyYourBreyer.com

International Museum of the Horse: IMH.org

North American Model Horse Shows Association: NAMHSA.org

The Horse Magazine: TheHorse.com/magazine

REFERENCES

American Museum of Natural History. "The Evolution of Horses." AMNH.org, 2019. AMNH.org/exhibitions/horse /the-evolution-of-horses.

Austin, Gloria. "Horses in History." EquineHeritageInstitute. org, July 22, 2013. EquineHeritageInstitute.org/horses -in-history.

Donoho, Emily. "Why Are Horses Measured in Hands? H&H Explains." *Horse & Hound*, December 26, 2017. HorseAndHound.co.uk/features/horse-measurement -hands-640677.

Equine Guelph. "How Horses See and Hear." University of Guelph, Ontario, Canada, n.d. EquineGuelph.ca/pdf /courses/trainer_kit/see_hear_notes.pdf.

Hayes, Karen. "Understand Your Horse's Eyesight." *Horse&Rider*, last updated April 22, 2020. HorseAnd Rider.com/horse-health-care/horse-vision-and-eyesight.

HorseAndMan.com. "Meet the World's Largest Horse (at That Time), Brooklyn Supreme!" *Horse & Man*, December 9, 2017. HorseAndMan.com/horse-stories /meet-worlds-largest-horse-time-brooklyn-supreme /12/09/2017.

Payne, Mike. "Glancing Back at History: Secretariat's Sprint into Immortality." *Beckett News*, Beckett Media LLC, May 20, 2018. Beckett.com/news/secretariat-1973 -belmont-stakes.

Reeve, Moira C. and Sharon Biggs. *The Original Horse Bible: The Definitive Source for All Things Horse: 175 Breed Profiles, Training Tips, Riding Insights, Competitive Activities, Grooming, and Health Remedies.* Irvine, CA: BowTie Press, 2011.

RoyRogers.com. "Trigger." RoyRogers.com, Accessed November 1, 2020. RoyRogers.com/trigger.

Savvy Horsewoman Equestrian Blog & Community. "Horse Sounds and Noises—What's Normal?" *Savvy Horsewoman*, May 9, 2019, SavvyHorsewoman.com /2019/05/horse-sounds-and-noises.html.

U.S. Department of Food and Agriculture. "Horse Senses." Cooperative Extension System, July 31, 2019. Horses.Extension.org/horse-senses.

Williams, Jennifer. "How to Read Your Horse's Body Language." EquusMagazine.com, Last updated October 5, 2020. EquusMagazine.com/behavior/horse-body-language.

ABOUT THE AUTHOR

Kelly Milner Halls adopted a wild mustang when she was 12 years old. Together, they learned how to be partners, and the

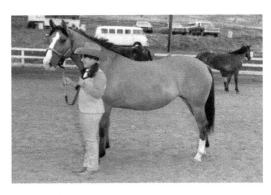

love never left her—even after she started writing nonfiction books for kids 20 years later. For more about those books, visit WondersOfWeird.com.

ABOUT THE ILLUSTRATOR

Jessie Willow Tucker grew up in Canberra, Australia, and completed a bachelor of fine arts degree at RMIT University in Melbourne and a post-graduate diploma in theater design at the Victorian College of the Arts. In addition to working as an illustrator, she has exhibited her fine art; worked in theater design, fashion design, and textile design; and managed her own fashion label.

CPSIA information can be obtained
at www.ICGtesting.com
Printed in the USA
JSHW040227091021
19413JS00001B/1